Table of Contents

Part 1: Introduction

Firstly, I would like to thank you all for reading my guide and I am sure that you will benefit from this guide given that you follow the instructions step by step. Secondly, I would like to tell you a bit about myself. My name is Nabel and I am an average college student. I like to consider myself a bodybuilder, however I am by no means a professional nor do I intend to make bodybuilding a profession. I am simply a passionate bodybuilder who has acquired knowledge through years of research and am passing it on to my fellow beginners.

I look up to a number of bodybuilders and seek their expertise for help, including Arnold Schwarzenegger, Ronnie Coleman, Branch Warren, and Jay Cutler. However, I am not interested in that 'huge bodybuilder look'. That is why I consider Aziz "Zyzz" Shavershian my ultimate idol (I am sure you have noticed his picture on the cover of this book), and my ultimate goal is to achieve his physique. He has motivated and inspired thousands of people to start a healthy lifestyle and to look after their physiques and he is the reason I began getting serious about bodybuilding and achieving the 'aesthetic' look.

The purpose of this guide is not to make you the number one bodybuilder or the world's strongest man, but it will lead you in the direction of achieving a great aesthetic physique and develop the strength required to develop such physique. I will give detailed explanations on diet and workout plans (including samples and examples) to help you achieve your goal. These methods are fool proof and will DEFINITELY work if you choose to follow ALL aspects of this guide and not only the ones that sound appealing you. Building an aesthetic physique is by no means an easy task and will require lots of patience, hard work, and dedication. If you are not willing to put in this effort, than I strongly advise you to stop wasting your time and close this book immediately. If it was easy, the average look would be an aesthetic one and we would all be aesthetic, but that is not the case at all.

One last thing before I get into the details. Do you know how all bodybuilding books out there bother explaining all the science behind the aspects they provide in their books that most of you probably will end up not understanding anyways? Well that is not my style as I prefer to get straight to the point. I will only give you information that is relevant to achieving that sexy aesthetic look. If you have reached this part, then congratulations, you have advanced to the next step. Get ready!

Part 2: Body Types

Every potential bodybuilder must know his body type before proceeding to tailor a diet/workout plan for himself. The reason for this is that there are different measures taken to achieve an aesthetic body for people who possess body types that are different. I will give you a brief outline on the three main body types; however I will refrain from going into excessive scientific detail that will simply put you to sleep and make you want to skip the invaluable parts of this book.

The three main body types are:

1) Endomorph: This body type is characterized as easily able to put on fat. It is also known for its difficulty in losing fat due to a slow metabolism that is caused by none other than a person's genetics. You may find people with endomorph-type bodies doing endless cardio, which isn't the exact solution to reaching the aesthetic level. A combination of

both cardio and weight lifting at the gym is more likely to shed the fat then doing boring hours of cardio alone. Very careful and measured dieting is the key to shedding the fat and revealing that aesthetic physique!

2) Mesomorph: This category is known for its ability to put on muscle easily. However, mesomorphs may also gain fat easily and/or lose muscle easily if diet is not carefully monitored. Mesomorphs appear broad and muscular though they may not have touched a weight in their lives due to favorable genetics, however to reveal a completely aesthetic physique a tailored diet and workout plan must be put into effect.

3) Ectomorph: This category is known for its extremely fast metabolism and difficulty packing on muscle (or even fat for that matter). In my opinion, this is the most difficult body type to deal with even though the ectomorph does not

have any fat to shed. A high calorie surplus is required of ectomorphs to build lean muscle. Do not get me wrong, however. You may hear people in this category telling you "I'm eating everything in sight to build muscle" only to see themselves ending up with a belly while maintaining their skinny physiques (these people are known as 'skinny-fat'). If it was as easy as consuming all the calories in the form of junk food then all ectomorphs would be lean and muscular, however a high calorie diet consisting of clean foods is required to pack on muscle for this specific body type.

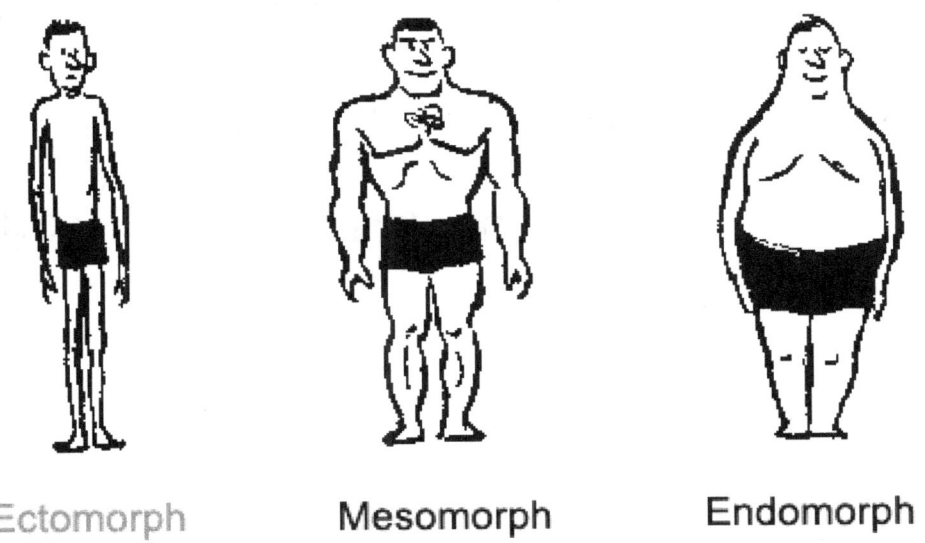

Ectomorph   Mesomorph   Endomorph

You may fall into one of these categories or the other, however many of us do not lie in any single one of these categories and may have picked up some of the traits of one body type and the rest of the traits from another. This is completely due to genetics and is out of our hands. For example, I would consider myself to be a meso-ectomorph. The reason for this is because I mainly possess the attributes of a mesomorph (easy ability to pack on muscle / easy ability to pack on fat), however I may have some characteristics of an ectomorph at the same time (slightly thin legs). Falling into any of these categories will not by any means prevent you from reaching that aesthetic physique you have been dying for. They all require hard work and dedication, and I am sure you will love the sport of bodybuilding and the lifestyle associated with it as much as I do!

Body Fat Percentage

You may have discovered your body type by now, but that information is not sufficient to tailor the perfect diet / workout to meet your specific needs. Body fat percentage is exactly what you need to work on finding out to know where your starting point lies. This percentage simply tells you the ratio of fat to total body weight you have in your body.

For the most accurate measurement of body fat percentage, I would recommend visiting your physician or local gym that may conduct body fat percentage tests using calipers. However, if you do not have access to these resources you may follow these steps carefully to determine your body fat percentage (may not be 100% accurate):

1) Measure your weight in pounds using any regular scale.

I will my own measurements for this example to make it

easier for you guys to follow. My weight in pounds is 172.

2) Multiply this number by 1.082 (172 x 1.082 = 186.104)

3) Add the result to 94.42 (186.104 + 94.42 = 280.524)

4) Measure your waist girth using any measuring tape you have around you at the belly button (navel) level. In my case, I measure at 29 cm.

5) Multiply your waist girth by 4.15 (29 x 4.15 = 120.35)

6) Subtract the number you have obtained in step 5 from the number you have obtained in step 3 (280.524 – 120.35 = 160.174). This number represents your lean body weight, which is what you would weight if you had no body fat at all (0% body fat percentage).

7) Finally, subtract your lean body weight from your actual body weight (found in step 1) and multiply the result by 100. Then, divide that result by your actual body weight.

To avoid confusion, your actual body weight has been used twice in this step

$172 - 160.174 = 11.826$

$11.826 \times 100 = 1182.6$

$1182.6 / 172 = $ **6.88% body fat**

That is how you measure your body fat ONLY if you are absolutely sure you have no access to a fitness center or clinic that can do it for you. The reason I say this is because the more accurate this percentage is, the more likely you are to plan a perfect-fitting diet / workout plan to achieve an aesthetic physique.

Below are simple guidelines to follow after you have determined your body fat percentage:

1) If you are under 10% body fat, you should follow a bulking diet with a constant caloric surplus consisting of clean foods and a workout a plan consisting mostly of resistance workouts and minimal cardio. You may incorporate cheat meals if you fall under this category (this will be discussed more in the diet section).

2) If you are between 10-14% body fat, you should follow a cutting/bulking diet (many may tell you that it is impossible to simultaneously bulk and cut, however I assure you from experience that it is very possible and I will explain my methods in the relevant sections of this book). You must also balance between cardio and resistance exercise if you fall under this category. Once you cut down to a single digit body fat percentage, you will start to follow the regimen of the first category.

3) If you are above 14% body fat, you should follow a cutting diet with a constant caloric deficit and focus heavily on cardio workouts and incorporate little resistance training (do not eliminate by any means). Once you cut down to a point where you fall in any of the two previous categories, then you pick up the regimen of that category.

Now that you know your body type as well as your body fat percentage, you should be well off and be ready to compose the perfect meal and workout plans to develop yourself into that ultimate aesthetic god you are aiming to be. The next step here is your diet plan, which definitely comes before your workout plan as you do know what they say: "muscles are made in the kitchen!"

Part 3: Diet

I cannot stress enough the importance of diet in a physique transformation, especially if you are aiming for the aesthetic look. In order to drop your body fat percentage to single digits and reveal that defined, chiseled body hiding underneath all that fat, you must be willing to be strict on yourself and measure everything you eat. I have a friend, Abraham, who is 'skinny-fat', or in other words, an ectomorph who believes eating anything in sight is the answer to gaining muscle mass. He also thinks that consuming alcohol a few times a week will not hinder his muscle building results. WRONG. As a result of his lack of attention to his diet, he now has a small belly forming onto his slim frame, therefore being pushed away from his goals. That is not what you are going to do. I will explain in the pages to come exactly how to tailor your diet so that you can pack on lean muscle and get shredded to reveal that aesthetic body of yours.

Three Main Food Groups

The three main macronutrients we consume in order to survive are carbohydrates, protein, and fats. We must focus on consuming all three of these groups in moderation to ensure a healthy lifestyle. Diet plans that ask you to completely eliminate one of these groups is bogus and will wear you out for no good reason.

1) Carbohydrates: There are two types of carbohydrates, complex and simple carbohydrates. Basically, we as bodybuilders must lessen our consumption of simple carbs and focus on getting our daily intake from complex carbs. Examples of both carbohydrates:

   a) Complex Carbohydrates: vegetables, fruits, beans, nuts, whole grain breads, brown rice, and wheat pasta

b) Simple Carbohydrates: white bread, sugar, fast food, soft drinks, confectionary

2) Protein: This is the macronutrient that we must focus on consuming no matter what our body type or body fat percentage is since it is the main muscle building block. Examples of high quality protein sources include: chicken breast, turkey breast, egg whites, fish, lean red meats, and low-fat (or skimmed) dairy products

3) Fats: This is the macronutrient that is considered highly debatable. The reason I say that is because many dieticians will advise their patients to avoid fats to lose weight. However, some fats are necessary in our lives and must be consumed to look aesthetic! These are known as unsaturated fats and omega-3 fats. However, other fats could actually set you back on your goals and prove to be

detrimental to your health, and these fats are known as saturated fats. Sources of these categories are:

a) Unsaturated Fats: nuts, avocado, olive oil, and vegetable oils

b) Omega-3 Fats: mackerel, salmon

c) Saturated Fats: whole-milk dairy, ice cream, poultry skin, cookies, cake, chips, and all of those snacks that you love!

Calorie Surplus v. Calorie Deficit

In terms of calories, you will be on one of these diets or the other: the calorie surplus diet or the calorie deficit diet. In the calorie surplus diet, you will be consuming more calories than your body burns throughout the day, therefore making your primary goal to build muscle (bulking). This diet is to be followed on all days for those of you who have body fat percentages under 10%.

As for the calorie deficit diet, it is the one where you must burn more calories than you consume, with a primary goal of fat loss (cutting). This diet is to be followed on all days for those with body fat percentages above 14%.

The tricky and most challenging choice is for those of you who lie in the 10-14% body fat percentage range. You are unsure whether to bulk or cut since you need to pack on a little muscle and lose a little more fat to reveal an aesthetic physique. Well, the answer is you have to do both at the same time! Many people will tell you that it is impossible to build muscle and lose fat at the same time (bulk and cut), however through a maneuver which I have personally tested myself and experienced, I learned that though it is not an easy task, it is definitely possible.

Carb Cycling / Zig-Zag Diet

The carb cycling / zig-zag diet is the answer to being able to simultaneously bulk and cut. The carb cycling concept of this diet is to follow a calorie surplus diet for certain days of the week (usually the days you train) and follow a calorie deficit diet on your rest days. The other 'zig-zag' concept of this diet is to consume a higher ratio of carbohydrates in comparison to protein and fats on surplus days while consuming a higher ratio of protein (and increase the fats a little) on deficit days. This causes your body to stay in shock mode, thus burning fat as you pack on lean muscle mass.

To be able to design a perfect diet for you, you must calculate your BMR (basic metabolic rate). The formula to find your BMR is as follows, and again I will use my measurements as an example to make it easier to follow (keep in mind weight is in pounds, height is in inches, and age is in years):

BMR = 66 + (6.23 x weight) + (12.7 x height) – (6.8 x age)

BMR = 66 + (6.23 x 172 lb) + (12.7 x 70 inches) – (6.8 x 19)

BMR = 66 +   1071.56   +   889   -   129.2

BMR = 1897 calories

Now, BMR isn't the final number we are looking for as it does not take into account a person's activity level. Since the exercise program I will have you follow involves you doing exercise 5-6 days a week, you should multiply your BMR by 1.7:

Calorie Needs = BMR x 1.7 = 1897 x 1.7 = 3,224 calories

Also, if you work at a job that requires you to do physical work all day long on top of your daily workouts, your calorie needs will be higher, therefore you are to multiply your BMR by 1.9 instead of 1.7:

Calorie Needs = BMR x 1.9 = 1897 x 1.9 = 3,604 calories

Now that you know your calorie needs, you will need to adjust that number according to your goal. If you are on a calorie surplus diet (bulking), I recommend adding 500-800 calories to that number and consuming that many calories every day. If you are on a calorie deficit diet (cutting), however, I recommend subtracting around 500 calories from your calorie needs and sticking to that number to shed the fat. I will include samples and make your lives easier in this chapter.

Water

The reason that I am dedicating a section specifically for water is its extreme importance for achieving an aesthetic physique. You must try and drink at least two gallons of water every day. The reason why you need to drink that much water is to avoid water retention and rid your body of the sodium cumulated in your muscles that gives them a bloated look. So before you ask, the answer is yes, drinking more water will help you get ripped. DRINK UP!

Meal Frequency

Remember your family tradition where you would eat three meals a day? Throw that concept out the window. You will now be eating smaller meals more frequently. Instead of eating three larger meals a day (breakfast, lunch, and dinner), you will be eating a meal every 2-3 hours if you are cutting or every 3-4 hours if you are bulking. The reason that meals are closer to each other in the cutting stage is because a fast for around 12-13 hours (a couple of hours before sleep, during sleep, and a couple of hours after waking up) where you would only drink water is beneficial for fat loss. Fasting is not required when on a bulk. Foods from each food group (protein, carbs, and fats) should be incorporated in every meal of the day.

Cheat Meals

There has been a long debate on the subject of cheat meals. Different opinions have been stated on this topic, with some people saying that occasional cheat meals are acceptable while others may say that cheat meals are detrimental to a bodybuilder's progress. In my opinion, the answer to this question depends on what stage of bodybuilding you are in. If you are in the first stage (over 14% body fat), I do not recommend cheat meals and actually strongly advise against them. If you are in the second stage (between 10-14% body fat), you may have one bi-weekly cheat meal (note that I said CHEAT MEAL and not CHEAT DAY). If you are in the third stage (below 10% body fat), you may have a weekly cheat meal or even maybe two cheat meals a week if you control them and keep them within your caloric requirements. A side note on cheat meals: DO NOT BINGE. Binge eating will set you back and hinder your progress. Plan your cheat meals in advance and ensure that you do not exceed your maximum caloric intake. Also, cheat days are completely unacceptable regardless of the stage you are in. If you want to develop an aesthetic appearance, cheat days are not for you. The only purpose of cheat meals is to satisfy a psychological craving and give your metabolism a little boost. Any more than a cheat 'meal' will have an adverse effect on your body and possibly even slow your metabolism down for a period of time.

Alcohol

Alcohol consumption is known to set back muscle growth. That is why professional bodybuilders stay away from alcohol and do not consume it regularly. We are not professional bodybuilders and that is why we may consume alcohol in moderation. I personally do not consume alcohol in order to avoid slowed progress completely; however a couple of drinks every other weekend will not set you back as much. Just make sure to choose liquor over beer since beer contains much more empty calories; and do not binge drink. A couple of drinks will do it if your tolerance is not that high due to infrequent drinking.

It is finally time to provide you guys with the sample diets you have been waiting for. You may change the contents of the diet around as long as you substitute them with foods of equal nutritional value and stick within the same ratios and calorie ranges. You should also make sure you are tailoring the amounts of the foods to your own personal caloric needs (which you have calculated in the previous section of this chapter). These diets are based on my calculations. Here are a few guidelines to follow if you are using my sample diets as templates:

1) If you are cutting (which you should be doing if you are above 14% body fat), then you should follow SAMPLE DIET 1 on all days of the week, be it a training day or a rest day.

2) If you are bulking (which you should be doing if you are below 10% body fat), then you should follow SAMPLE

DIET 2 on all days of the week, be it a training day or a rest day.

3) If you are unsure on whether to bulk or cut (between 10-14% body fat), then you should alternate both diets so that you are following a 'zig-zag' diet. Therefore, you would be following SAMPLE DIET 1 on rest days to be in a caloric deficit and you would follow SAMPLE DIET 2 on training days so that you are in a caloric surplus. This will allow you to gradually and efficiently out on muscle mass while shedding fat.

Finally, before moving on to the sample diets, I have included the suggested supplements to be used while following each sample diet. Refer to the supplements chapter in this book to look up the function of each supplement.

SAMPLE DIET 1 for 170 lb male (CALORIC DEFICIT)

Wake Up Meal (8:00 AM):

- 1 Acetyl-l-Carnitine
- 1 tall glass of water
  TOTAL: 0 calories, 0g carbs, 0g protein, 0g fat

Breakfast (10:00 AM):

- 2 eggs
- 2 egg whites
- ¼ cup low fat mozzarella cheese
- ½ large-sized whole wheat pita bread
- 2 fish oil capsules
- 1 multi vitamin capsule
- 1 zinc capsule
- 1 vitamin D3 capsule
- 1 vitamin C capsule
  TOTAL: 468 calories, 21g carbs, 37g protein, 26g fat

Pre-Workout (12:00 PM):

- 2 BCAA capsules
  TOTAL: 0 calories, 0g carbs, 0g protein, 0g fat

Post-Workout (2:00 PM):

- 2 scoops whey protein
- 8 oz reduced fat milk
- 1 tbsp natural peanut butter
- 1 vitamin C capsule
  TOTAL: 447 calories, 19g carbs, 58g protein, 15g fat

Lunch (4:00 PM):
- 8 oz chicken breast
- 3 oz zucchini
- 1 cup cooked whole wheat rice OR whole wheat pasta
- 1 tbsp natural peanut butter
- 1 COD liver oil capsule
- 1 multi vitamin capsule
  TOTAL: 704 calories, 45g carbs, 83g protein, 21g fat

Dinner (7:00 PM):

- 8 oz chicken breast
- 3 oz zucchini
- 1 cup cooked whole wheat rice OR whole wheat pasta
- 1 tbsp natural peanut butter
- 1 COD liver oil capsule
- 1 magnesium capsule
- TOTAL: 704 calories, 45g carbs, 83g protein, 21g fat

30 minutes before bed (10:00 PM)

- 1 melatonin capsule
- 3 ZMA capsules
  TOTAL: 0 calories, 0g carbs, 0g protein, 0g fat

TOTALS OF SAMPLE DIET 1

2,323 calories
130g carbs
261g protein
83g fat

SAMPLE DIET 2 for 160 lb male (CALORIC SURPLUS)

Wake Up Meal (8:00 AM):

- 1 tbsp honey
- 1 scoop whey protein
- ½ tsp micronized creatine powder
- mix all in 8 oz water
  TOTAL: 174 calories, 19g carbs, 23g protein, 1g fat

Breakfast (10:00 AM):

- protein pancakes (mix 2 oz egg whites, 1 egg, 2 oz oats, 1.5 scoops whey protein and cook on stove with 1 tsp butter)
- 1 serving sugar free maple syrup
- 1 digestive enzyme capsule
- 1 multi vitamin capsule
- 1 vitamin C capsule
  TOTAL: 576 calories, 49g carbs, 55g protein, 19g fat

Pre-Workout (12:00 PM):

- ½ tsp micronized creatine powder
- pre-workout supplement
- mix all in 6 oz water
  TOTAL: 37 calories, 9g carbs, 0g protein, 0g fat

Post-Workout (2:00 PM):

- 12 oz 100% grape juice
- 1 scoop whey protein
- ½ tsp micronized creatine powder
- 1 vitamin C capsule
  TOTAL: 410 calories, 65g carbs, 23g protein, 1g fat

Lunch (4:00 PM):

- 10 oz chicken breast
- 2 cups cooked whole wheat pasta OR whole wheat rice
- 6 oz chunky Ragu tomato sauce
- green tea mixed with 1 tbsp honey
- 1 digestive enzyme capsule
- 1 multi vitamin
  TOTAL: 1,124 calories, 131g carbs, 112g protein, 16g fat

Snack (6:30 PM):

- 1 cup reduced fat Chex Mix
  TOTAL: 200 calories, 31g carbs, 2g protein, 7g fat

Dinner (9:00 PM):

- 10 oz chicken breast
- 2 cups cooked whole wheat pasta OR whole wheat rice
- 6 oz chunky Ragu tomato sauce
- 1 digestive enzyme capsule
- 1 magnesium capsule
  TOTAL: 1,091 calories, 114g carbs, 112g protein, 16g fat

Pre-Bed Meal (11:00 PM):

- 8 oz reduced fat plain yogurt
- 1 tbsp honey
- 1 scoop whey protein
- ¼ cup pineapple chunks
  TOTAL: 358 calories, 43g carbs, 36g protein, 5g fat

TOTALS OF SAMPLE DIET 2

3,970 calories
461g carbs
363g protein
65g fat

Part 4: Training

A Few Words on Weight Lifting

Weight lifting forms the base of an aesthetic body. You will not be able to achieve an aesthetic physique without lifting weights, no matter what people tell you. Endless ab exercises alone will not give you a great set of abs. You must train every muscle in your body to achieve your goals. Improving the muscularity of your chest, for example, will not come along without training your triceps. You must tailor your workout plan to exercise each and every muscle.

Training for Strength v. Training for Mass

Lifting weights in order to gain mass cannot be achieved without making strength gains. The reason for this is because when you get stronger and lift heavier weights, your muscles will be forced to adapt to this heavier weight load by increasing in size. Therefore, if you do not gain strength, you will not gain mass. The difference in training to make strength gains than training to make mass gains is the rep range of your workouts. Strength gains rely on heavier weights in the low rep range (3-5 reps) while mass gains rely on weights you can do in the 8-12 rep range. The solution to make BOTH strength and mass gains simultaneously is to mix both low rep workout days with high rep workout days in your workout program. I found the best routine as having one upper body strength day (low reps), one lower body strength day (low reps), and three hypertrophy training days (focus on specific muscles and consist of high rep exercises) throughout the week. This will be shown in more detail in the sample workout section.

Pushing Yourself to the Limit

Should you push yourself to the extreme limit when lifting weights? Absolutely. That final rep that you did with extreme difficulty will not have gone in vain, I promise. It will definitely pay off and that last extra rep is the one that will tell your muscle that it needs to grow to be able to adapt to the heavier weight exerted on it. What I do to keep my muscles lifting heavier is record every single rep I do at the gym on my phone so that when I do the same exercise the following week, I'll slightly increase my weight and force myself to lift that weight to keep growing and avoid reaching a plateau. I would also refrain from repeating the same exact exercises and routine every week as repetitive workouts may cause a plateau, so I usually set up two different workout plans for myself, training the same muscle groups, and alternate them every other week.

Cardio

Different cardio workouts are effective in helping you lose fat; however doing endless cardio workouts is not the answer to developing an aesthetic body. Setting up a meal plan and following that meal plan religiously makes up at least 70% of your progress, and training makes up the other 30%. While bulking, I personally do not do any cardio at all. Walking to school or work if it is close by rather than taking the bus or driving is enough cardio for me while on a bulk since many hard earned calories are lost through cardio. If you are cutting, however, cardio is encouraged and should be done 2-3 times a week (preferably directly after weight training). High intensity interval training (HIIT) has been proven to be the best form of cardio. HIIT will be explained in more detail in the next section.

High Intensity Interval Training (HIIT)

This is the only type of cardio that has worked wonders for me and allowed me to drop to a single digit body fat percentage. You do not have to perform this exercise for more than 20 minutes each time and it gives you much better results than long hours wasted on the treadmill. The beauty of HIIT is that you can use it for any form of cardio. The example I am giving here of an HIIT routine is my treadmill running routine, here is how it's done:

- 4 minutes warm-up (6 mph)

- 30 second high intensity (12 mph)

- 60 second moderate intensity (8 mph)

- 45 second high intensity (12 mph)

- 60 second moderate intensity (8 mph)

- 60 second high intensity (12 mph)

- 60 second moderate intensity (8 mph)

- 90 second high intensity (12 mph)

- 60 second moderate intensity (8 mph)

- 60 second high intensity (12 mph)

- 60 second moderate intensity (8 mph)

- 45 second high intensity (12 mph)

- 60 second moderate intensity (8 mph)

- 30 second high intensity (12 mph)

- 4 minutes cool-down (6 mph)

TOTAL TIME TAKEN = 20 MINUTES

Simply put, in less time you can achieve better results. HIIT cardio is the way to go and it will have you shredded given that you follow a set meal plan to accompany it while on your cutting phase. Do not do this routine more than 3 times a week though, especially if you are lifting weights as well. This cardio will have you fatigued if you overwork yourself.

Exercises

This is a guide to all the exercises I recommend doing to gaining lean muscle and reaching your aesthetic goal. I will categorize the exercises according to muscle group and will include sample workout routines following this section. Enjoy!

Back:

1. Barbell Row

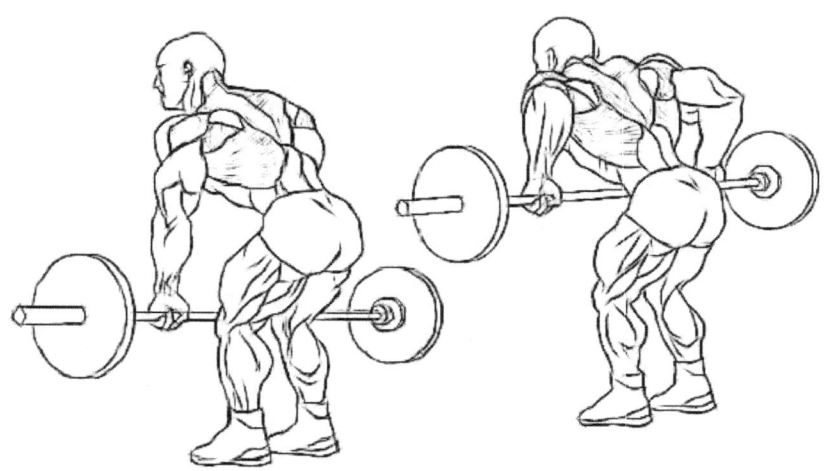

2. Deadlift

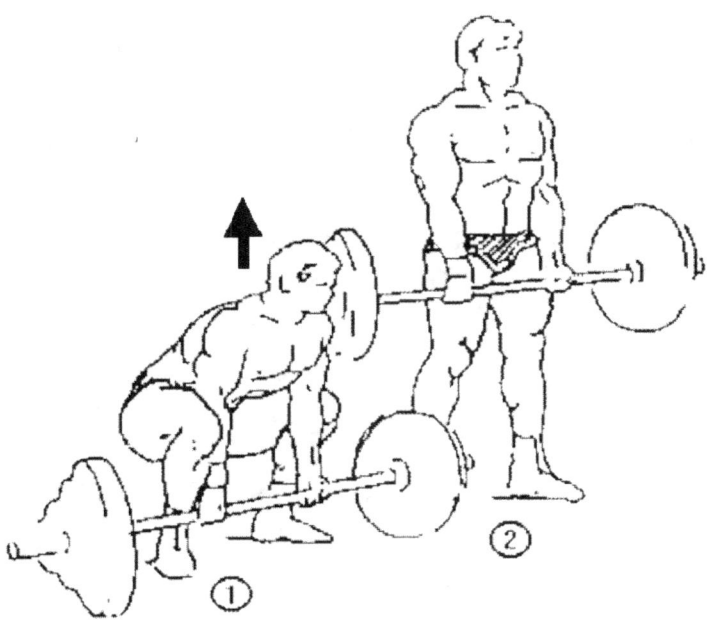

3. Weighted Wide-Grip Pullup

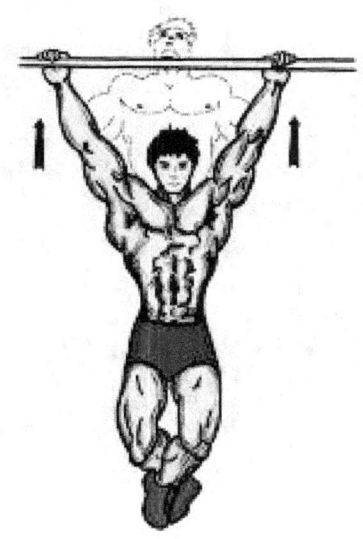

4. Wide-Grip Lat Pulldown

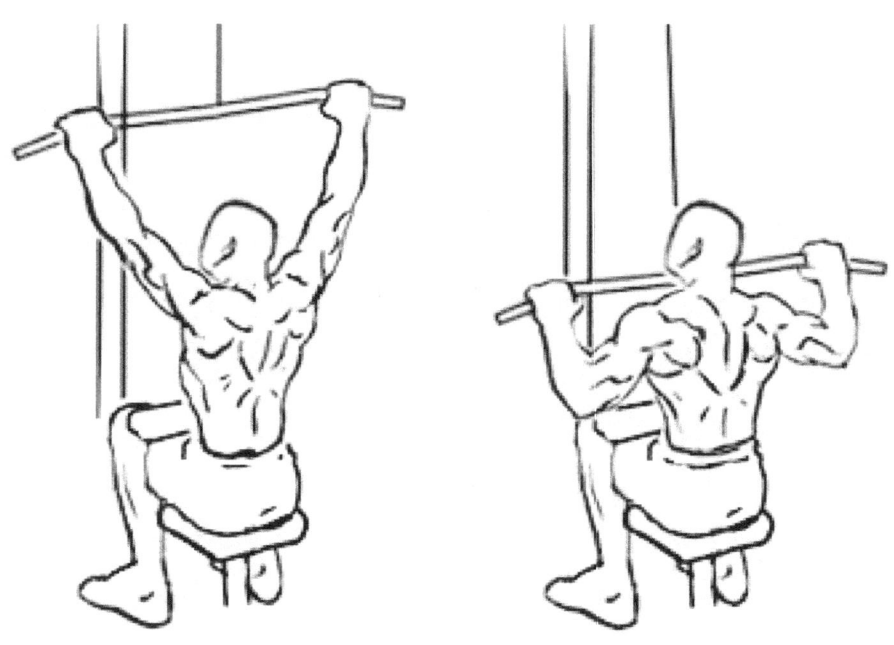

5. Rack Chins

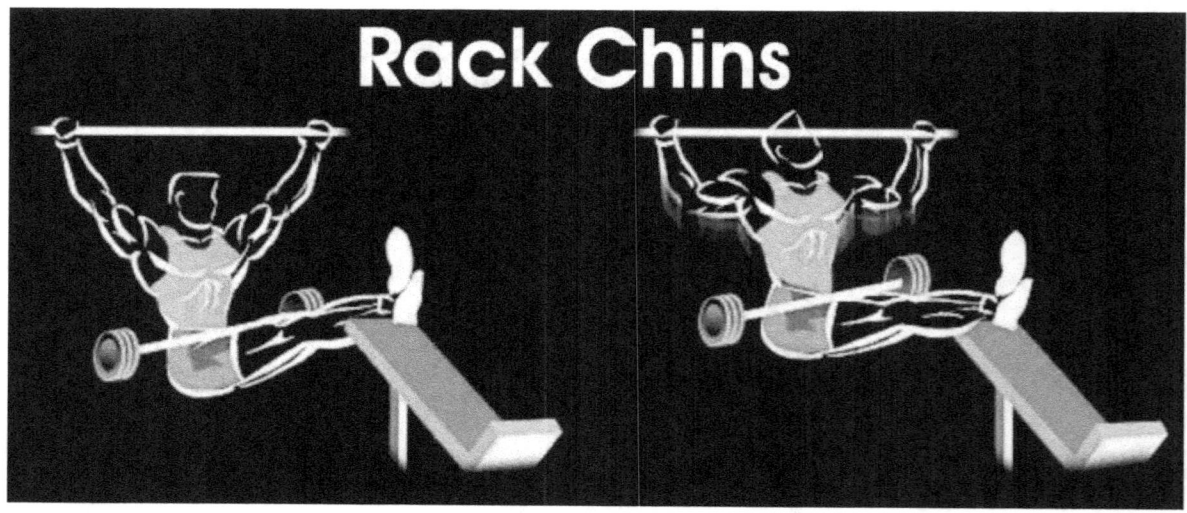

6. Machine Row

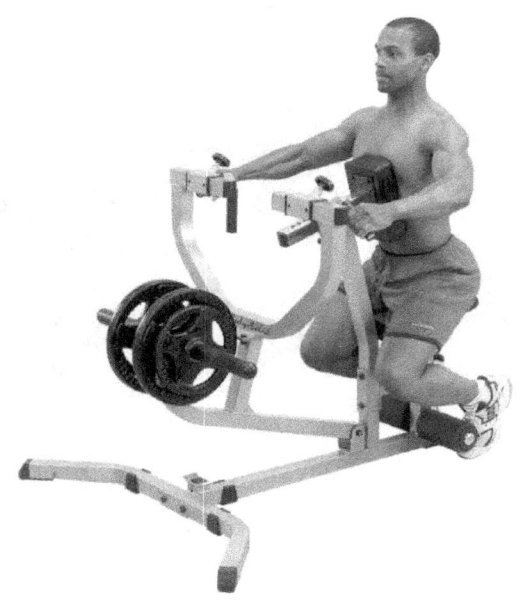

7. Seated Cable Row

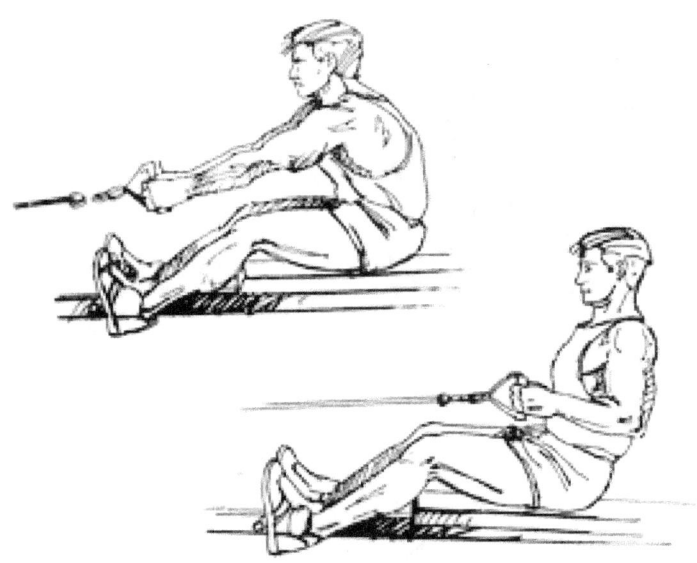

8. Dumbbell Rows on Incline Bench

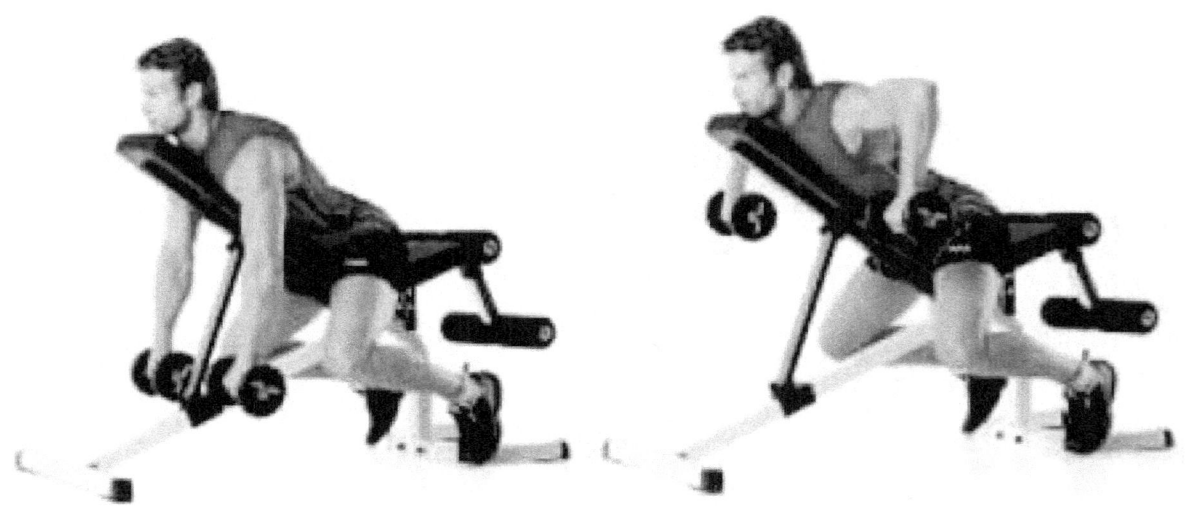

9. Bent Over Dumbbell Row

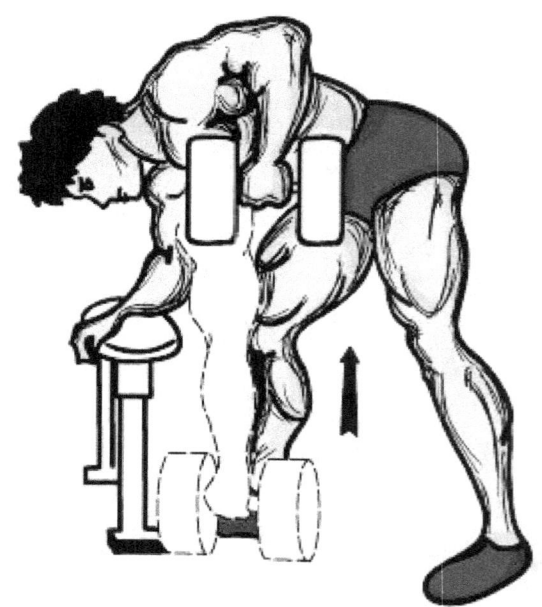

10.   Close-Grip Pulldown

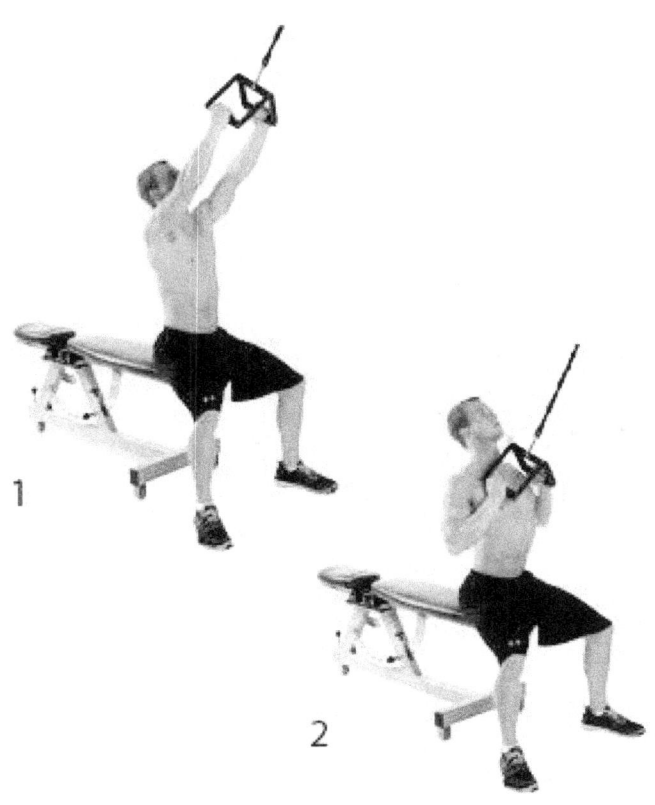

Chest:

1. Bench Press

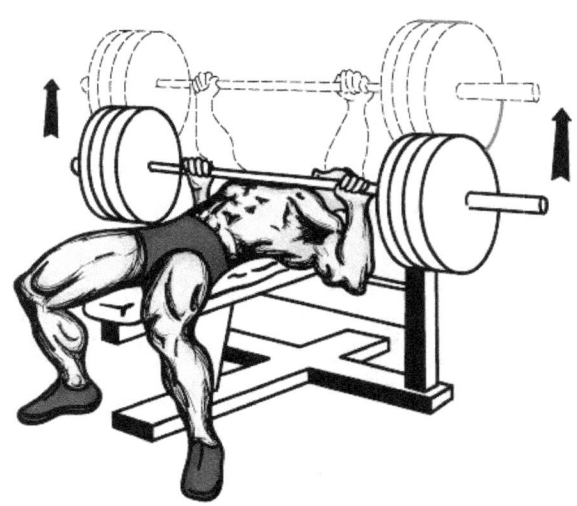

2. Flat Dumbbell Press

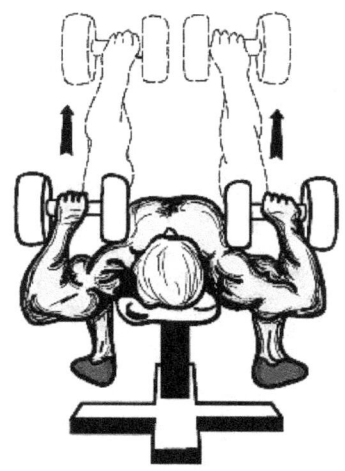

3. Chest Dips

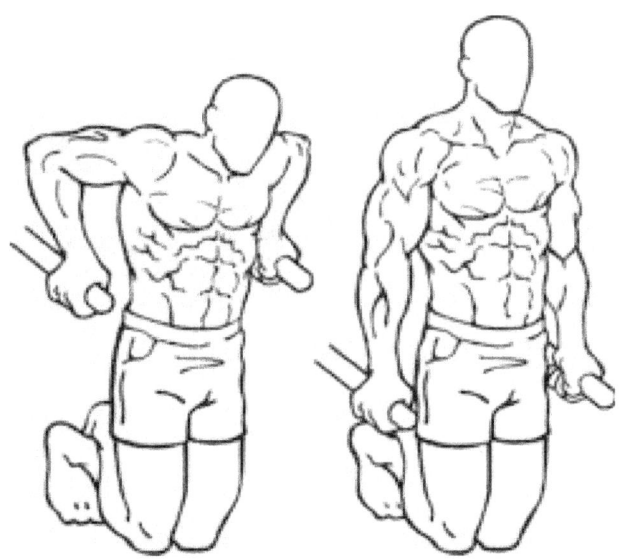

4. Incline Bench Press

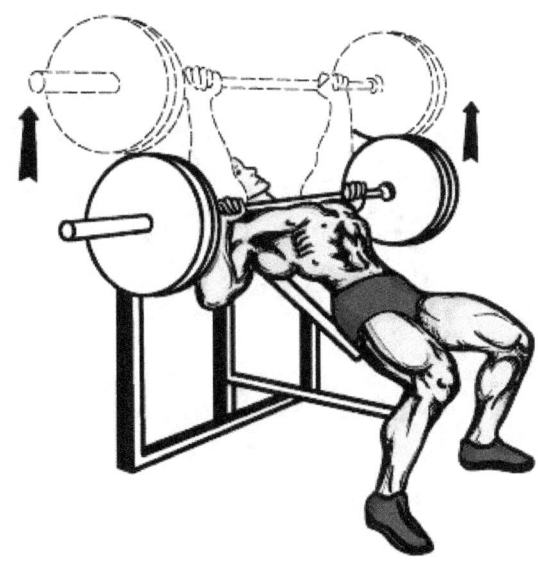

5. Incline Dumbbell Press

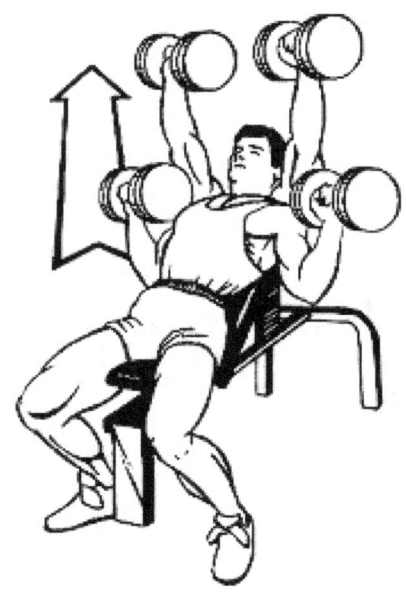

6. Machine Chest Press

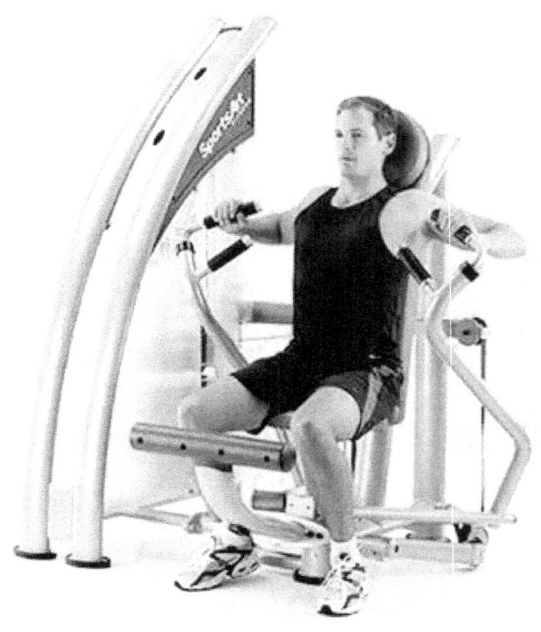

7. Machine Flyes

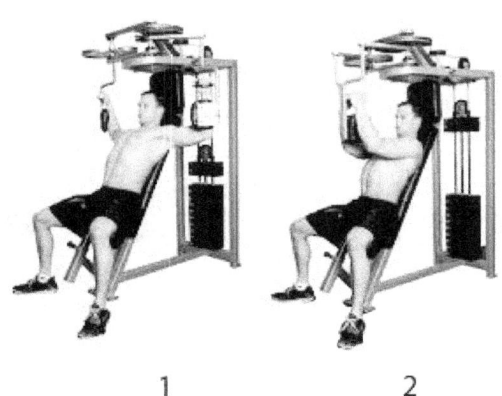

1   2

8. Incline Flyes

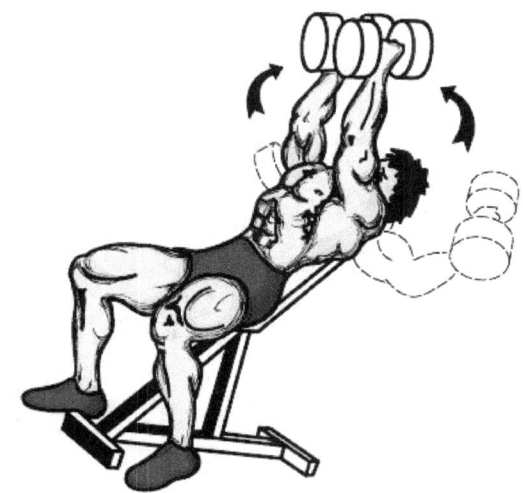

Shoulders:

1. Dumbbell Shoulder Press

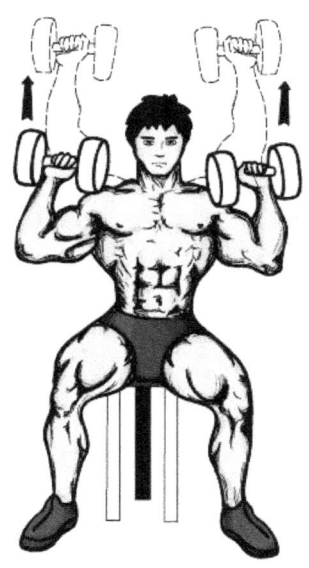

2. Military Press

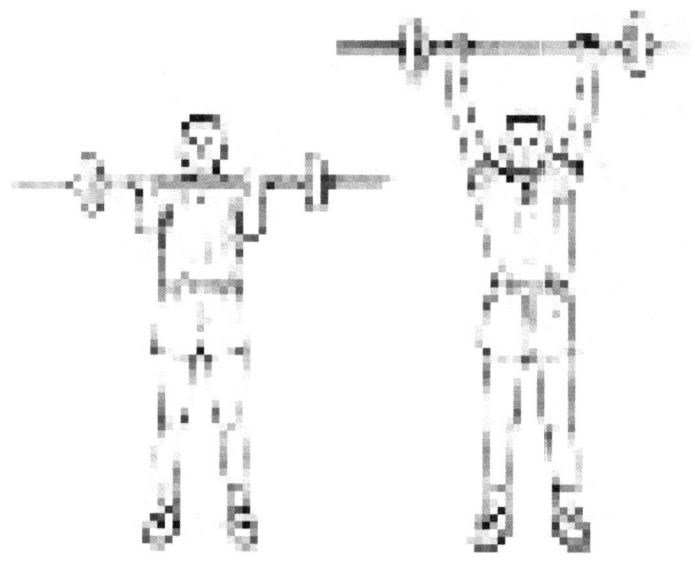

3. Upright Rows

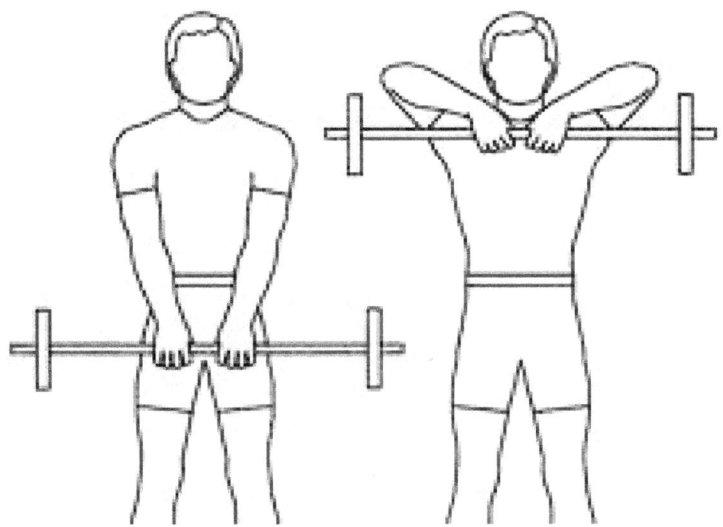

4. Side Lat Raise

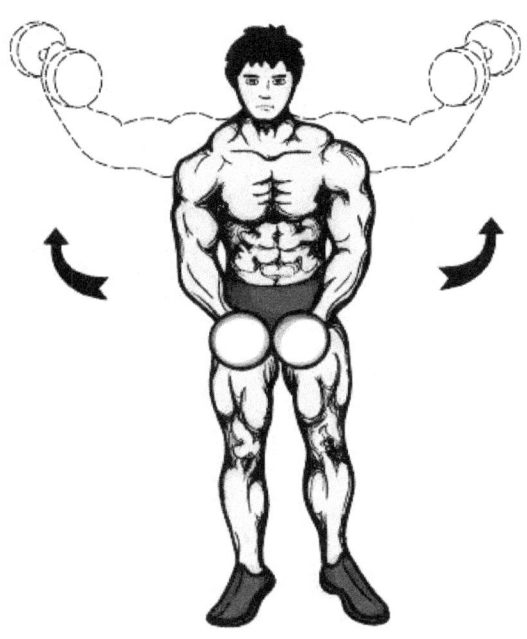

5. Front Lat Raise

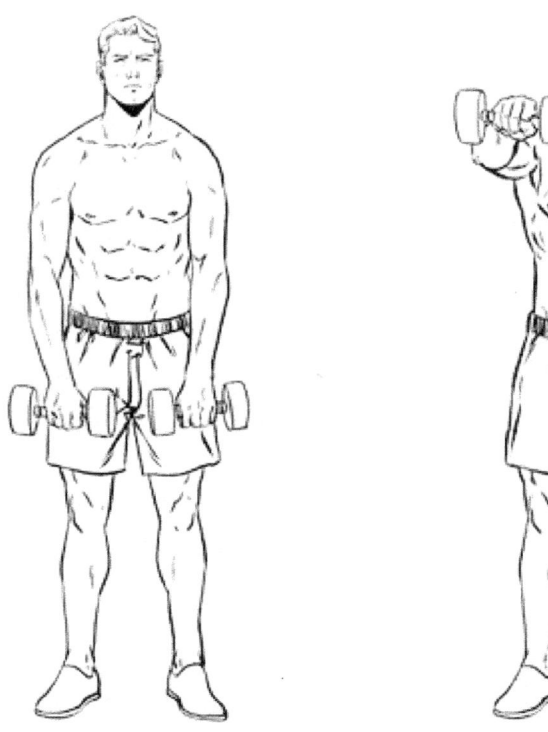

Biceps:

1. Barbell Curl

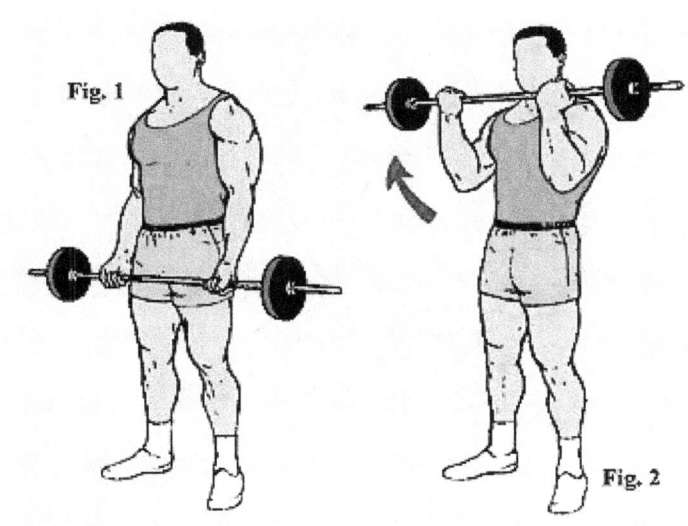

Fig. 1

Fig. 2

2. Dumbbell Curl

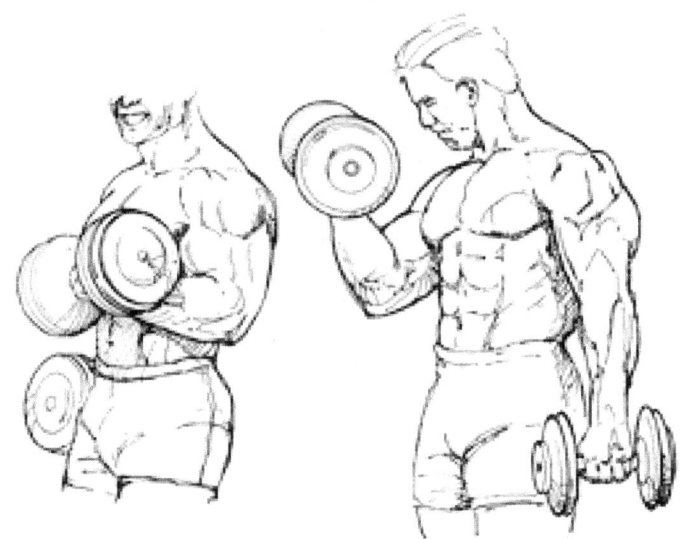

3. Preacher Curl

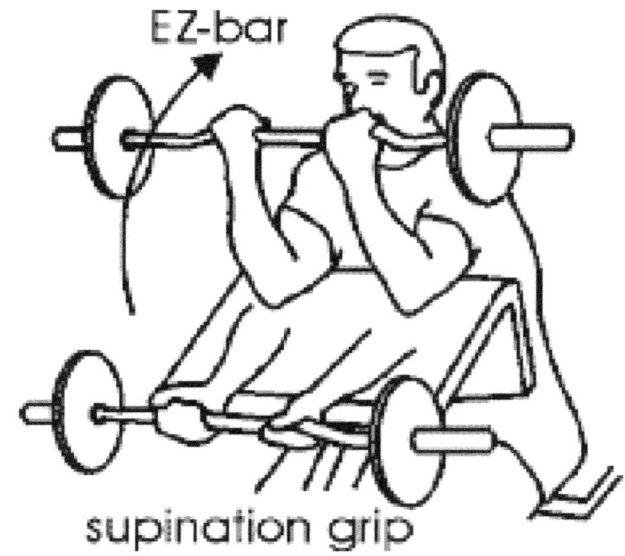

EZ-bar

supination grip

4. Concentration Curl

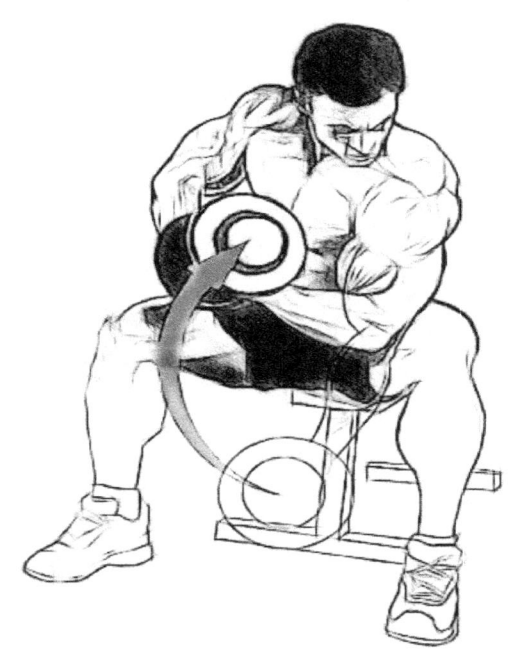

5. Spider Curl

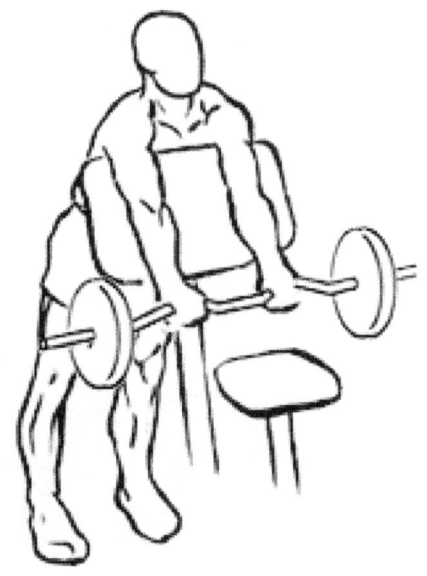

6. Hammer Curl

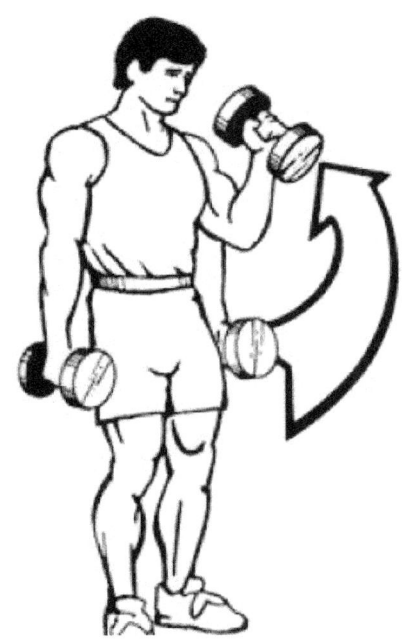

Triceps:

1. Skull Crusher

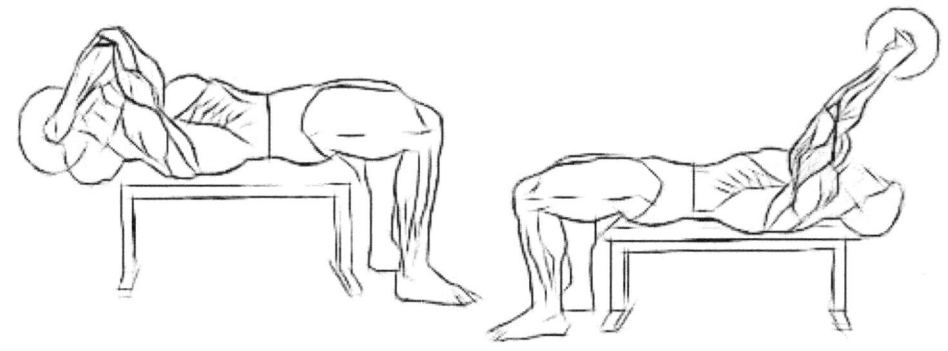

2. Tricep Extension

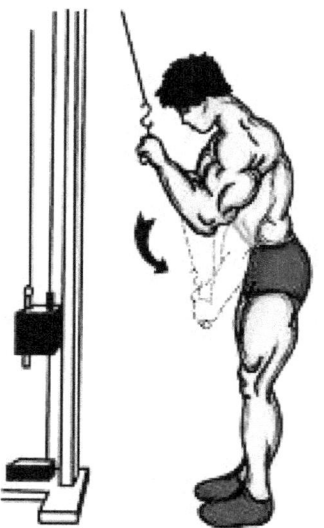

3. Standing Dumbbell Tricep Extension

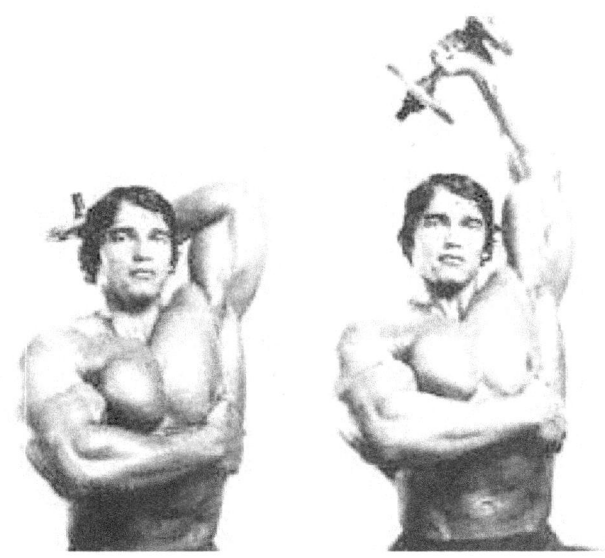

4. Rope Tricep Extension

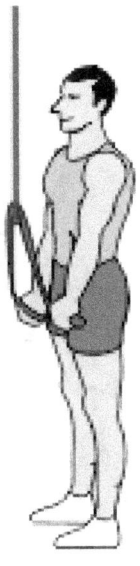

5. Cable Kickback Tricep Extension

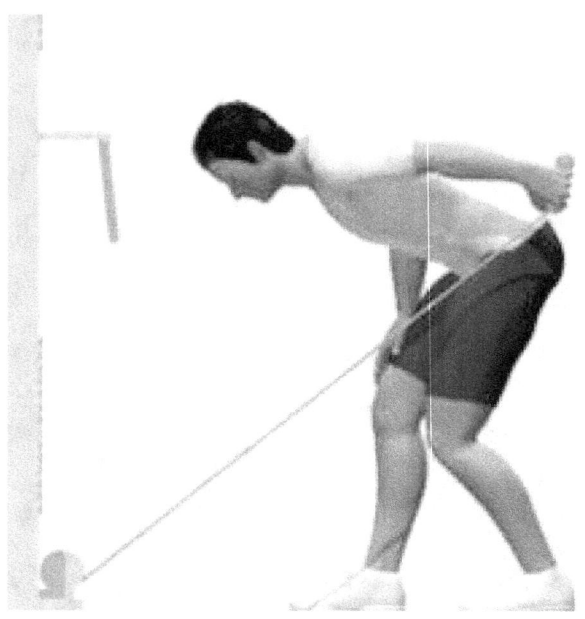

6. Overhead Rope Tricep Extension

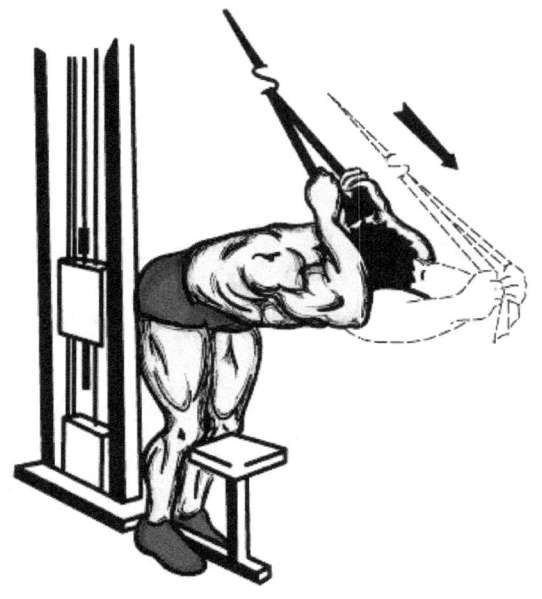

Legs:

1. Barbell Squats

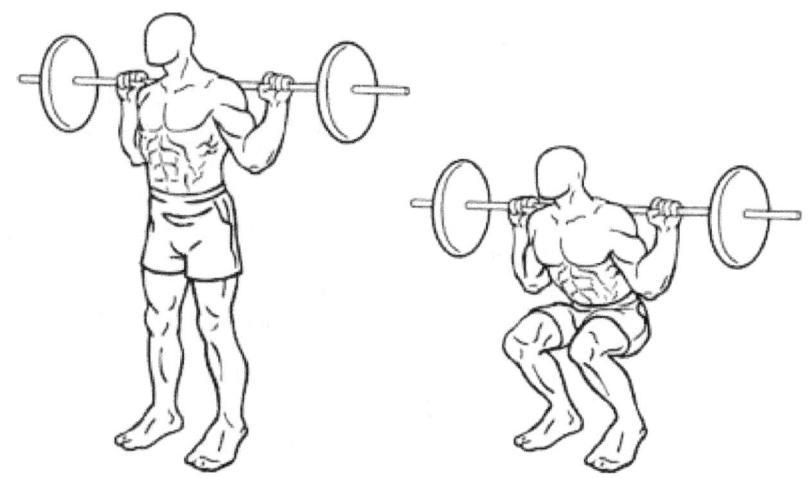

2. Dumbbell Squats

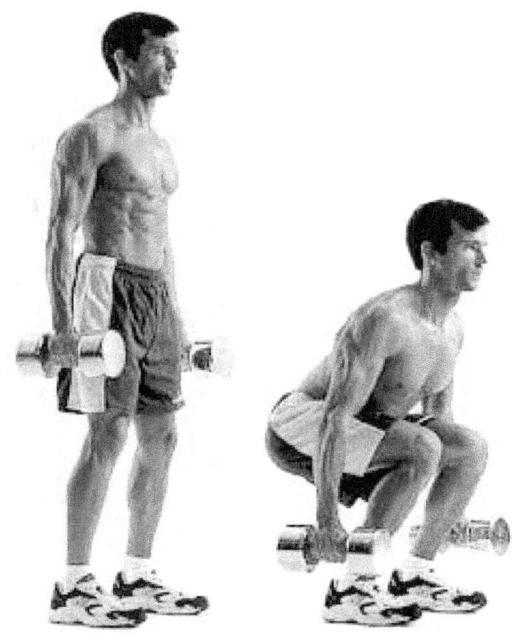

3. Leg Press

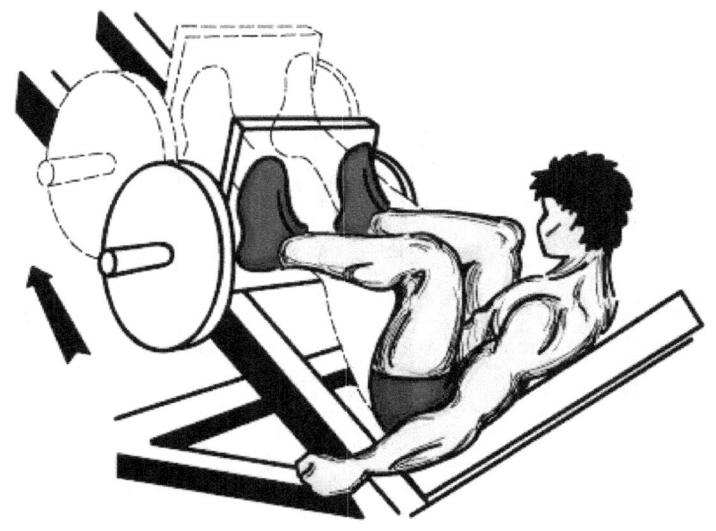

4. Leg Extension

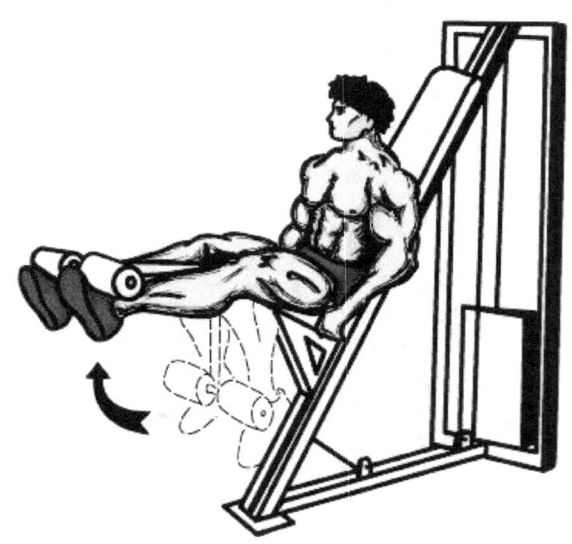

5. Stiff-Leg Deadlift

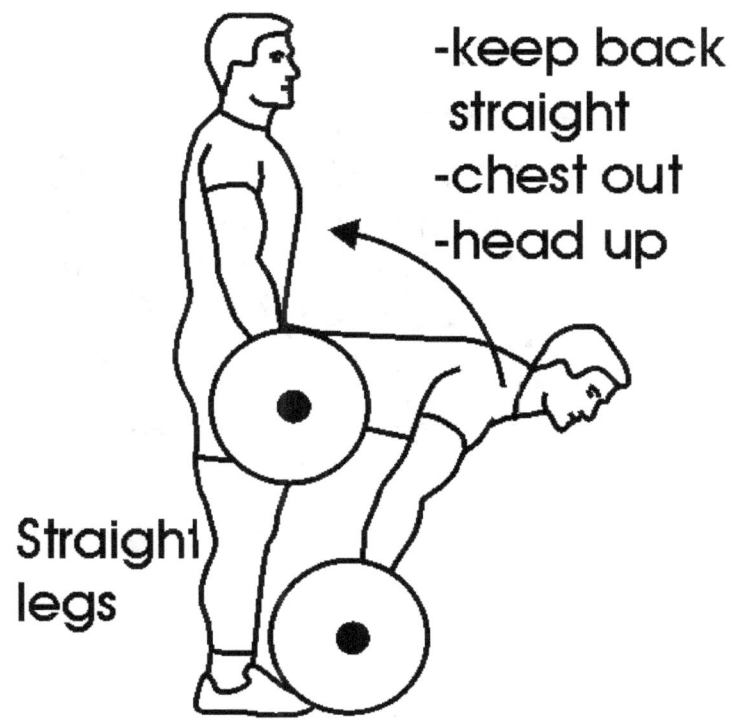

-keep back
 straight
-chest out
-head up

Straight
legs

6. Seated Leg Curls

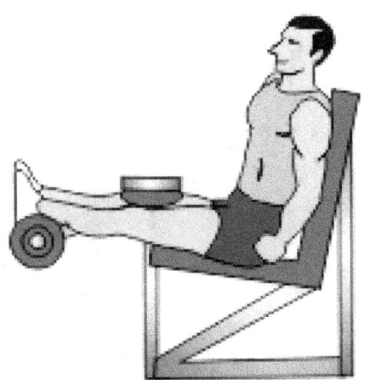

7. Lying Leg Curls

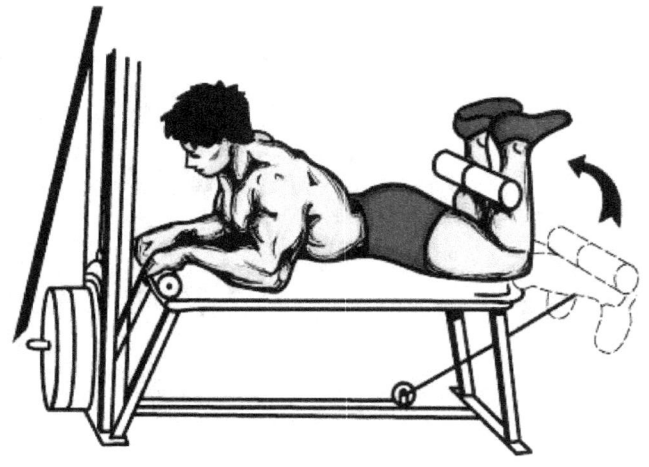

8. Standing Calf Raise

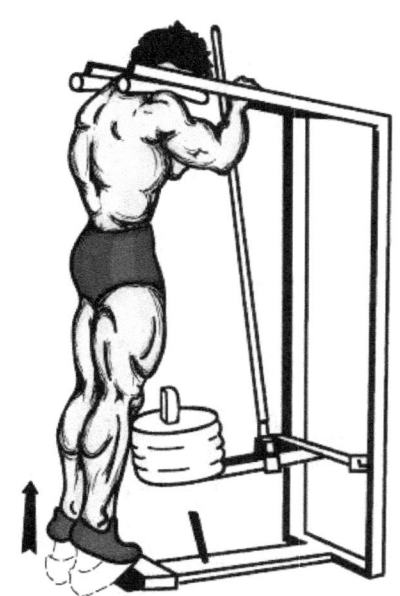

9. Seated Calf Extension

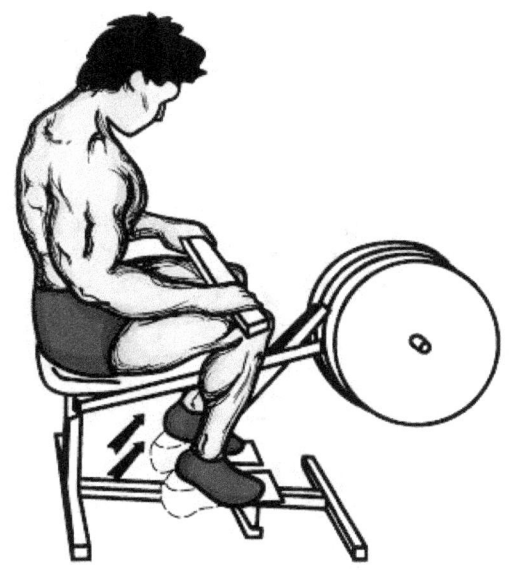

Abs:

1. Cable Crunch

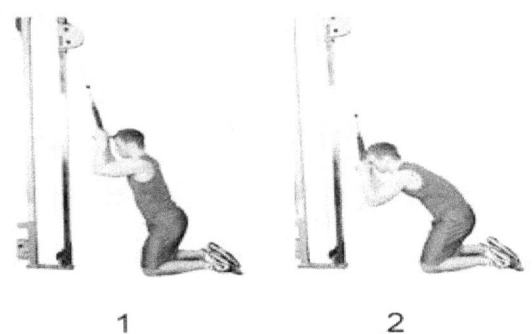

1   2

2. Decline Weighted Crunch

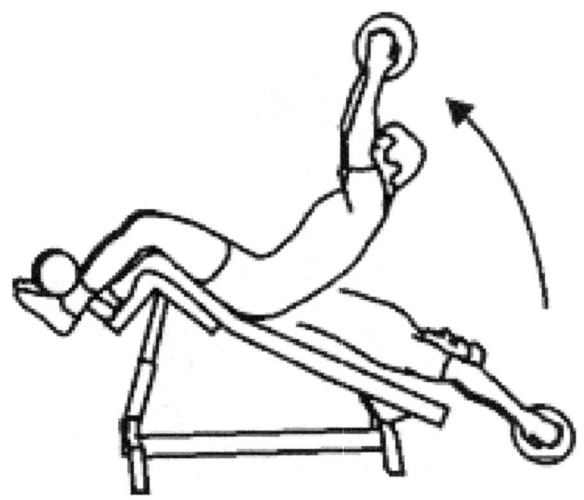

3. Hanging Leg Raise

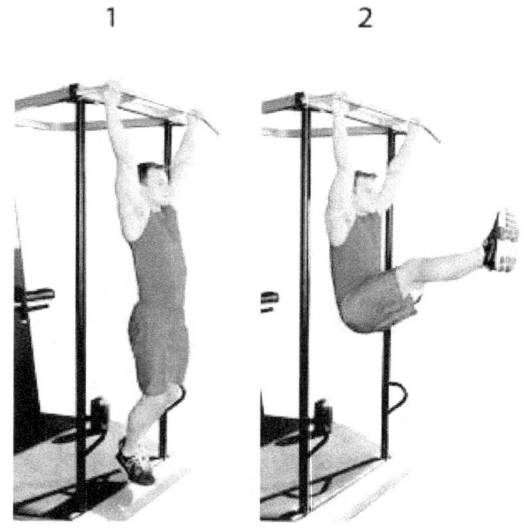

4. Hanging Leg Raise to Side

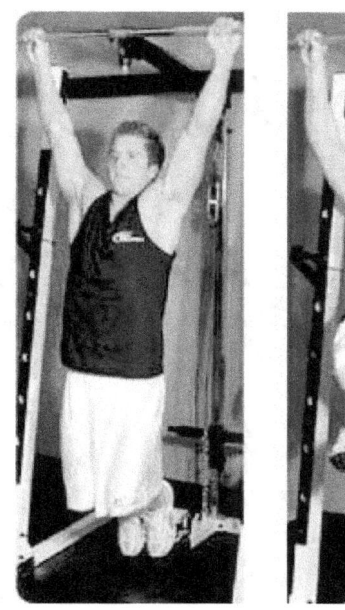

5. Flat Bench Crunch

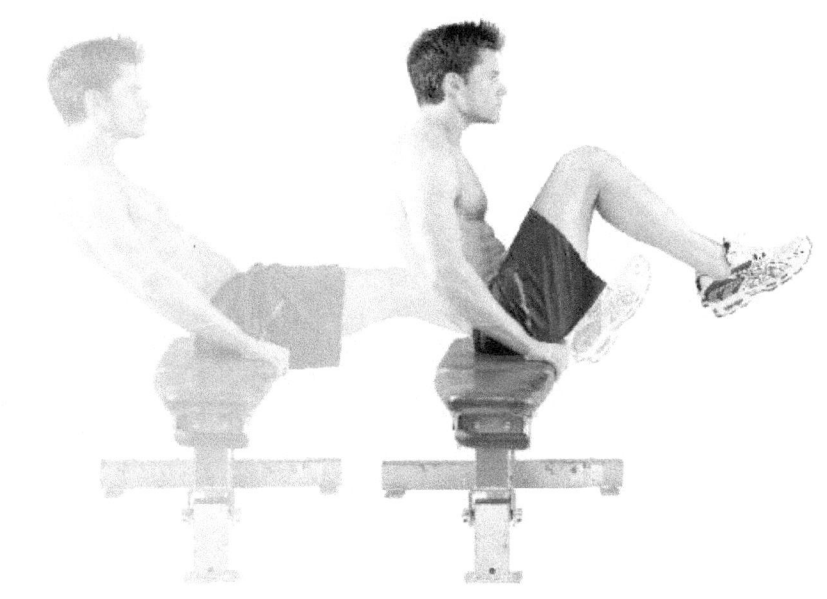

6. Double Crunch

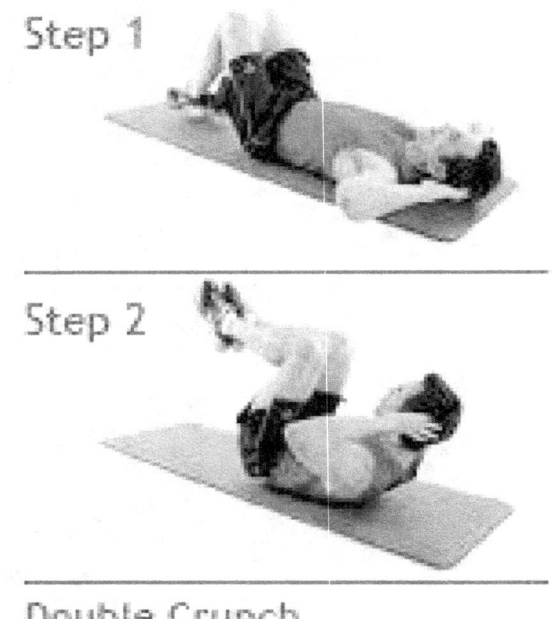

Step 1

Step 2

Double Crunch

7. Plate Twist

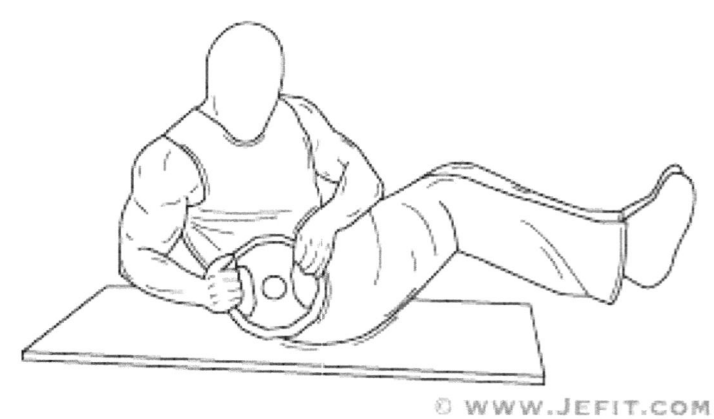

© WWW.JEFIT.COM

---

8. Dumbbell Side Bend

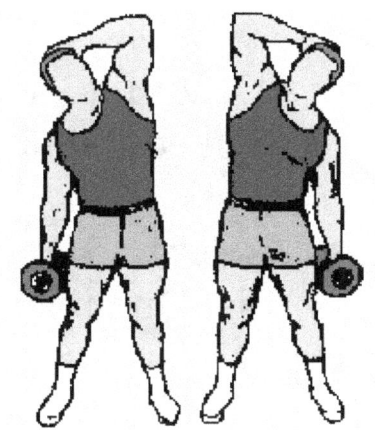

Now that you have all of the exercises under your belt, here is a sample workout routine that will definitely help you achieve an aesthetic physique, given that you follow a suitable diet plan for your body type of course! Wherever you see the symbol "/", you may alternate the mentioned workouts to avoid a plateau in muscle growth. Enjoy!

SAMPLE WORKOUT ROUTINE

Monday (Upper Body Strength):
- Barbell Row / Deadlift (3 sets x 5 reps)
- Wide-Grip Weighted Pullup / Wide-Grip Pulldown (2 sets x 6-10 reps)
- Rack Chins (2 sets x 6-10 reps)
- Bench Press / Flat Dumbbell Press (3 sets x 3-5 reps)
- Weighted Dips (2 sets x 6-10 reps)
- Shoulder Press / Military Press (3 sets x 6-10 reps)
- Barbell Curl / Dumbbell Curl (3 sets x 6-10 reps)
- Skull Crushers / Tricep Extension (3 sets x 6-10 reps)
- Decline Weighted Crunches (3 sets x 8-12 reps)
- Hanging Leg Raises (3 sets x 10-12 reps)
- Double Crunch (3 sets x 8-12 reps)
- Dumbbell Side Bends (3 sets x 8-12 reps)

Tuesday (Lower Body Strength):
- Barbell Squats (3 sets x 3-5 reps)
- Leg Press (2 sets x 6-10 reps)
- Leg Extension (2 sets x 6-10 reps)
- Stiff Leg Deadlift (3 sets x 5-8 reps)
- Seated Leg Curls / Lying Leg Curls (2 sets x 6-10 reps)
- Standing Calf Raise (3 sets x 6-10 reps)
- Seated Calf Extension (2 sets x 6-10 reps)

Wednesday (REST if BULKING / HIIT if CUTTING)

Thursday (Back & Shoulders Mass Building):
- Barbell Rows / Deadlift (6 sets x 3 reps)
- Rack Chins (3 set x 8-12 reps)
- Machine Row / Seated Cable Row (3 sets x 8-12 reps)
- Dumbbell Rows on Incline Bench / Bent Over Dumbbell Row (2 sets x 12-15 reps)
- Close-Grip Pulldown (2 sets x 15-20 reps)
- Shoulder Press / Military Press (3 sets x 8-12 reps)
- Upright Rows (2 sets x 12-15 reps)
- Side Lat Raises / Front Lat Raises (3 sets x 15-20 reps)

Friday (Chest, Biceps, Triceps, & Abs Mass Building):
- Bench Press / Flat Dumbbell Press (6 sets x 3 reps)
- Incline Bench Press / Incline Dumbbell Press (3 sets x 8-12 reps)
- Chest Press / Machine Flyes (3 sets x 12-15 reps)
- Incline Flyes (2 sets x 15-20 reps)
- Barbell Curl / Preacher Curl (3 sets x 8-12 reps)
- Concentration Curl (2 sets x 12-15 reps)
- Spider Curl / Hammer Curl (2 sets x 15-20 reps)
- Tricep Extension / Dumbbell Tricep Extension (3 sets x 8-12 reps)
- Rope Tricep Extension / Tricep Extension (2 sets x 12-15 reps)
- Cable Kickback / Overhead Tricep Extension (2 sets x 15-20 reps)

Saturday (Legs & Abs Mass Building):
- Barbell Squats (6 sets x 3 reps)
- Dumbbell Squats (3 sets x 8-12 reps)
- Leg Press (2 sets x 12-15 reps)
- Leg Extension (3 sets x 15-20 reps)
- Stiff Leg Deadlift (3 sets x 8-12 reps)
- Seated Leg Curls / Lying Leg Curls (4 sets x 15-20 reps)
- Standing Calf Raise (4 sets x 10-15 reps)
- Seated Calf Extension (3 sets x 15-20 reps)
- Cable Crunch (3 sets x 8-12 reps)
- Hanging Leg Raise to Side (3 sets x 10-12 reps)
- Flat Bench Crunch (3 sets x 8-12 reps)
- Dumbbell Side Bend (3 sets x 8-12 reps)

Sunday (REST if BULKING / HIIT if CUTTING)

Part 5: Supplementation

Supplements are known to be helpful towards achieving one's muscle building or fat loss goals. However, we should remember that supplements are not the most important part of our diets and we should only use them to help us achieve our goals and not rely on them to miraculously make us appear aesthetic. Here is an overview on the supplements used in the diet part of this book:

1. Whey Protein: this type of protein powder digests quickly and is high in amino acids, which is crucial for muscle recovery.

   Recommended Brand: ON's Gold Standard 100% Whey

2. Micronized Create Powder: a supplement that gives you that extra boost you need to finish that last rep. This supplement has been highly debated and thought to have

negative effects on its users, however, THESE THOUGHTS ARE FALSE. Creatine is actually very beneficial in bodybuilding and does wonders for you if used in moderation. Just remember to drink lots of water especially when using creatine to avoid water retention in your body!

Recommended Brand: ON's Micronized Creatine Powder

3. Multi-Vitamins: This supplement provides essential vitamins, minerals, and other crucial nutrients to our body. It is also important for our energy levels, performance, and vitality.

Recommended Brand: ON's Opti-Men

4. Vitamin C: an antioxidant vitamin that could help reduce risk of certain forms of cancer.

Recommended Brand: NOW's C-500

5. Digestive Enzyme: essential to the body's absorption and full use of food. Contains different enzymes to ensure digestion of all types of macronutrients.

Recommended Brand: Life Extension's Digestive Enzymes

6. Pre-Workout Supplement: this supplement gives you energy to pump you up for your workout. It is to be taken around 30 minutes before you start your workout.

Recommended Brand: BSN's N.O. Xplode

7. Magnesium: a supplement that is essential for calcium and potassium assimilation. Magnesium aids in proper nerve muscle impulses, enzyme reactions, formation of bone and carbohydrate metabolism, anxiety, and nervousness.

   Recommended Brand: Twinlab's Magnesium Caps

8. Cod Liver Oil: a fish oil supplement rich in vitamins A and D and Omega-3 fatty acids.

   Recommended Brand: NOW's Cod Liver Oil Capsules

9. Acetyl-L-Carnitine: an amino acid that supports cellular energy production. This supplement should be taken on a cutting diet first thing in the morning on an empty stomach.

   Recommended Brand: NOW's Acetyl-L-Carnitine

10. Fish Oil: this supplement is a great source of Omega-3 fatty acids. The human body does not manufacture fish oil, thus it must be supplemented. They are necessary for rebuilding existing cells and the production of new cells.

    Recommended Brand: ON's Fish Oil Softgels

11. Zinc: a valuable and natural mineral for optimum health

    Recommended Brand: Ultimate Nutrition's Zinc

12. Vitamin D3: vitamin D is a key vitamin and essential for strong bones, dental health, and structural support

    Recommended Brand: NOW's Chewable Vitamin D-3

Part 6: Rest

You may be thinking why there is a chapter solely dedicated to the topic of 'rest'. The reason I have done this is the extreme importance of rest to a bodybuilder. Without adequate amounts of rest, muscles will not be able to recover, thus causing fatigue and inability to train. You must get at least 8 hours of sleep every night. If you cannot get your 8 hours of sleep during the weekdays, push for at least 6 hours and make up for the lost sleep on the weekends.

Overtraining is another important factor that must be highly considered. Training a muscle group more than twice a week will cause your muscles to wear out and fatigue, thus hindering muscle growth. You should also avoid training the same muscle groups two days in a row. Many people make the mistake of doing ab workouts every day. Abs should not be done on consecutive days and not more than twice a week.

Part 7: Music

To make your bodybuilding experience as glorious and great as mine, I am going to provide you with my music playlist to recommend some tracks to listen to during your workouts. If you do not have a taste for trance music, DO NOT CONTINUE.

This playlist consists completely of trance music, here goes:

1. Blow Me – DJ D
2. I Wish It Could Last (Hook and Sling Remix) – Sam La More
3. Only a Few Things – Above & Beyond ft Zoe Johnston
4. Sun Moon Marcus Schossow Remix - Above & Beyond t Richard Bedford
5. Can't Sleep (Radio Edit) - Above & Beyond
6. Anphonic (Arty Remix) – Above & Beyond
7. Doing It Right Original Mix – Afrojack
8. Take Over Control – Afrojack ft Eva Simmons
9. Brain Leech (Bugged Mind Remix) – Alex Gopher
10. Better Off Alone – DJ Jurgen
11. Never Say Never (Omnia Remix) – Armin Van Buuren
12. As Above, So Below (Justice Remix) – Klaxons
13. Holding Me Kissing Me (FNP Remix) – Colours ft Domino
14. Never Cry Again – Dash Berlin
15. My Direction (Dougal & Gammer Remix) – D-Code
16. Arguru (EDX's 5un5hine Remix) – Deadmau5
17. I Remember (Original Mix) – Deadmau5
18. Elements – Dinka
19. Sweet Love (Lambretto Remix) – Disco Superstars

20. Eurodance – DJ Mangoo
21. Set Me Free (DJ Neo Short Cut) – DJ Session One
22. Century (ft Calvin Harris) – Tiesto
23. Somebody (Leventina Remix) – DJ Tatana
24. She Gave Happiness (Arty Remix) – D-Mad
25. Feel the Power – D-Mix
26. We Are Rockstars (Cold Blank Remix) – Does It Offend
27. Over (Rokonix Remix) – Drake
28. Stranger to Stability (Len Faki Podium Mix) – Dustin Zahn
29. Easy Muffin – Amon Tobin
30. Stereo Love (Massivedrum & DJ Fernando Hit Mix 2010) – Edward Maya
31. Electric Feel (Justice Remix) – MGMT
32. Sweet Dreams (Nick Corline Remix) – Eurythmetics
33. Nobody Said it was Easy – Evil Activities
34. Let Me Be Real (Radio Edit) – Fedde le Grand
35. Cream (Arcade Remix) – Federico Franchi
36. My Sanctuary – First State
37. Reverie (ft Sarah Howells) – First State
38. The Sacrifice – Headhunterz
39. Hyper Trance Hymn – Yoji Biomehanika
40. Big Sky (Agnelli & Nelson Remix) – John O'Callaghan
41. Find Yourself (Original) - John O'Callaghan ft Sarah Howells
42. Take It All Away (Marcus Schossow Mix) – John O'Callaghan
43. Wet n Wild – K.I.M.
44. Angel On My Shoulder (EDX Remix) – Kaskade
45. My World (Original Mix) – Kill the Noise
46. Use Somebody (Armin van Buuren Remix)
47. Amsterdam (Smith & Pledger Remix) – Luminary

48. Chasing Love – Maor Levi
49. The New World - Markus Schultz
50. No Good (Original Mix 2005) – Max B. Grant
51. You & I (Deadmau5 Remix) – Medina
52. Kids (Soulwax Remix) – MGMT
53. On the Surface (Alex M.O.R.P.H. Remix) – Mike Shiver
54. Trentemoller Remix – Modeselektor
55. Shana (Duderstadt Progressive Dub Mix) – Mr. Pit
56. Beachball – Nalin & Kane
57. Beachball 2010 (DBN Remix) – Nalin & Kline
58. This Moment (Prog Mix) – Nic Chagall
59. Morning Light (Remix) – Nic Chagall
60. True Rebel – Nitrogenetics
61. No Turning Back (Original Mix DRM) – Gui Boratto
62. Wonderless (Monster Mix) – Oasis vs Myon
63. Remember the Name – Osiris
64. Pump It Up (CJ Stone Atmosphere Mix) – Potatoheads
65. Monster (Camo & Crooked Remix) - Professor Green ft Example
66. I Wish It Could Last (Hook & Sling Remix) – Sam La More
67. For the Most Part (Marcus Schossow Remix) – Sean Tyas
68. Kidsos (Wippenberg Remix) - Sebastian Ingrosso
69. Imprisoned – Shogun
70. Cool (Afrojack Remix) – Spencer & Hill
71. One (Your Name) (Original Mix) – Swedish House Mafia
72. One (ft Pharell) – Swedish House Mafia
73. The Moment It Breaks -Tydi ft Tania Zygar
74. Trinity – Ummet Ozcan
75. Alpha (Original Mix) - W&W

76. King of My Castle 2009 (Rowald Steyn Remix) - Wamdue Project
77. Faces (Original Mix) – Andy Moor
78. Must Have Been a Dream (Original Mix) – Drax and Scott Mac
79. Deep Down (Alex M.O.R.P.H. Remix) – Josh Gabriel
80. Helpless (Monster Mix) – Myon & Shane
81. Winter – DT8 Project
82. No One On Earth (Gabriel and Dresden Remix) – Above & Beyond
83. Faithfulness – Skin
84. Blue Fear – Armin Van Buuren
85. Alone Tonight (Original Mix) – Above & Beyond
86. Always Besides Me (Club Mix) – Sandee
87. Beautiful Things (Gabriel & Dresden Remix) – Andain
88. New York City – Armin Van Buuren
89. Burned with Desire (Rising Star Remix) – Armin Van Buuren
90. Yet Another Day – Armin Van Buuren
91. Corrupted - Signal Runner
92. Say Hello – Deep Dish
93. Madras (In Search of Sunrise) – Tiesto
94. Twelve – Tiesto
95. Find – Ridgewalkers
96. Free Fallin – Claudia Cazacu
97. Haunted – Lo-Fi Sugar / Paul Van Dyk
98. I Am What I Am – Above & Beyond
99. Into the Sea (Moonrise Edit) – CJ Stone
100. Ordinary Day (MDE Mix) – Judge Jules
101. Just Be – Tiesto
102. Life is too Short (Energy Mix) – Kai Tracid

103. Love Comes Again (Radio Edit) – Tiesto
104. My World (Arksun Remix) – Luminary
105. Mind of the Wonderful – Blank & Jones
106. Southern Sun (Solar Stone Chill Out Mix) – Paul Oakenfold
107. La Noche – Tiesto ft Coca & Villa
108. Nothing At All (ft Rex Mundi) – Susana
109. Silence – Delerium
110. Summerfish (Scandall Sunset on Ibiza Mix) – Leonid Rudenko
111. Talk Like a Stranger (Markus Schulz Remix) – Armin Van Buuren ft Deepsky
112. Tell Me – Tiesto
113. Walking On Clouds – Tiesto
114. Karen Overton – Your Loving Arms

Part 8: Conclusion

This is the end of it, folks! We've covered everything from daily caloric needs, body fat percentage, custom-tailored diet plans, custom-tailored workout routines, and supplements.

It's not going to be easy adapting to the bodybuilding lifestyle, since you will have to commit to a training routine as well as adapt your eating habits to meet the requirements of the bodybuilding life. I would just like to encourage you to stay encouraged and do not give up. Results do not happen overnight and you must be patient and keep yourself motivated throughout the whole process.

For any bodybuilding questions or inquiries on how to achieve an aesthetic body, feel free to email me at khatutn@gmail.com